Sirtfood Diet

The Ultimate Cookbook With

Easy and Tasty Recipes

Melissa Clark

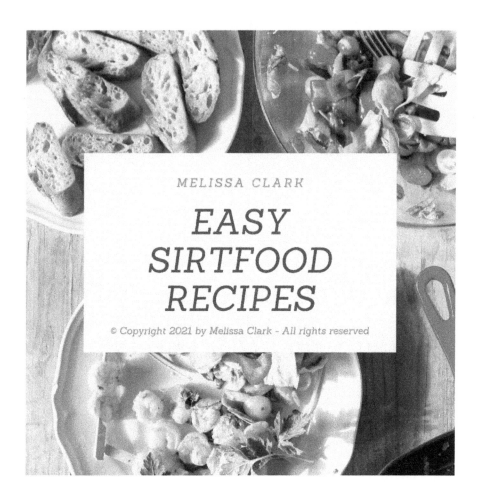

MELISSA CLARK

EASY SIRTFOOD RECIPES

Table of Contents

MELISSA CLARK
HAPPY COOKING
New Recipes
Sirtfood Diet
© COPYRIGHT 2021 BY MELISSA CLARK – ALL RIGHTS RESERVED

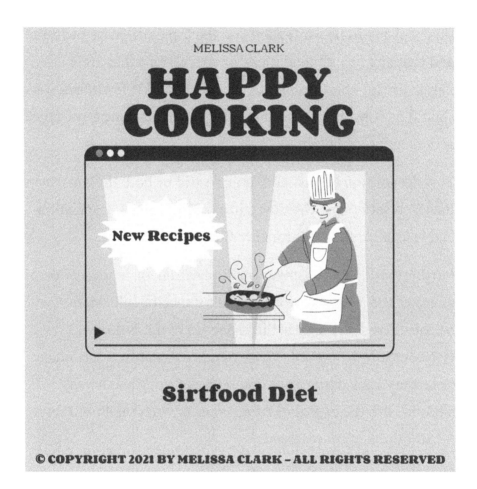

The information in the following pages is broadly considered a truthful and accurate account of facts and as such, any inattention, use, or misuse of the information in question by the reader will render any resulting actions solely under their purview. There are no scenarios in which the publisher or the original author of this work can be in any fashion deemed liable for any hardship or damages that may befall them after undertaking information described herein.

Additionally, the information in the following pages is intended only for informational purposes and should thus be thought of as universal. As befitting its nature, it is presented without assurance regarding its prolonged validity or interim quality. Trademarks that are mentioned are done without written consent and can in no way be considered an endorsement from the trademark holder.

INTRODUCTION

This diet relies on research sirtuins (SIRTs), a set of seven proteins utilized from the human anatomy that's been proven to modulate various purposes, including inflammation, metabolism, and life span.

Certain Natural plant chemicals could find a way to grow the degree of those proteins inside the human anatomy, and foods containing them are known "sirtfoods."

The diet blends sirtfoods and calorie limitation, both of which may cause the human body to generate high degrees of sirtuins.

The Sirtfood Diet publication comprises meal plans and recipes to follow along; however, there are lots of additional Sirtfood diet recipe books out there.

The diet's founders claim that a Sirtfood Diet can cause accelerated body weight loss while maintaining muscles and protecting you from chronic illness.

When your own body is energy-deprived, it melts away its catastrophe energy stores, or glycogen, along with burning off muscle and fat.

Each Molecule of glycogen necessitates 3--4 atoms of water to bestow. Whenever your body melts away glycogen, then it eliminates the water too. It's referred to as "water."

The very first week of extreme calorie limit, just about one-fifth of that fat loss arises from fat, whereas one other two-thirds stems out of water, glycogen, and muscle.

When your calories grow, the own body accomplishes its glycogen stores, and also, the weight comes back again. Regrettably, such a calorie restriction may also cause the human body to reduce its metabolism, which makes it need fewer calories every day for energy compared to previously. Additionally, a diet might likely help you drop a couple of pounds at the start, although it is going to probably return once the diet has ended.

The Sirtfood Diet contains 2 stages. About all the first few days, you just drink three 'sirt juices' and also have just one meal (full of 1000 calories each day). Over the subsequent four days, you are allowed two sirt juices along with 2 meals per day (full of 1,500 calories per day). Then you advance to the much easier phase 2, together with one juice along with also three 'balanced' meals, in thoughtful portion sizes, daily.

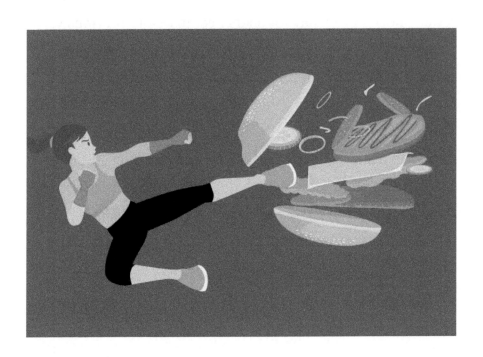

BREAKFAST

Prawn & Chili Pak Choi

Preparation Time: 30 minutes

Cooking Time: 15 minutes

Servings: 1

Ingredients:

- 75g brown rice
- 1 pak choi
- 60ml chicken stock
- 1 tbsp extra virgin olive oil
- 1 garlic clove, finely chopped
- 50g red onion, finely chopped
- ½ bird's eye chili, finely chopped
- 1 tsp freshly grated ginger
- 125g shelled raw king prawns
- 1 tbsp. soy sauce
- 1 tsp five-spice
- 1 tbsp. freshly chopped flat-leaf parsley
- A pinch of salt and pepper

Directions:

1. Bring a medium sized saucepan of water to the boil and cook the brown rice for 25-30 minutes, or until softened.

2. Tear the pak choi into pieces. Warm the chicken stock in a skillet over medium heat and toss in the pak choi, cooking until the pak choi has slightly wilted.

3. In another skillet, warm olive oil over high heat. Toss in the ginger, chili, red onions and garlic frying for 2-3 minutes.

4. Throw in the pawns, five-spice and soy sauce and cook for 6-8 minutes, or until the cooked throughout. Drain the brown rice and add to the skillet, stirring and cooking for 2-3 minutes. Add the pak choi, garnish with parsley and serve.

Nutrition: Calories: 403 kcal Protein: 16.15 g Fat: 15.28 g Carbohydrates: 50.87 g

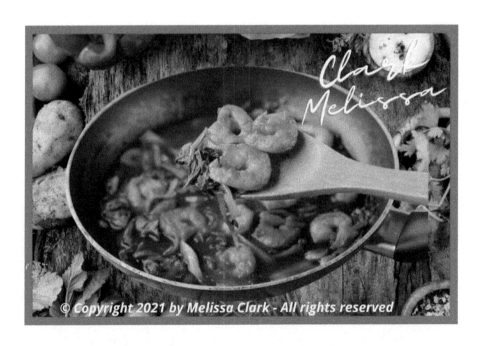

Sirtfood Granola

Preparation Time: 1 hour 10 minutes

Cooking Time: 50 minutes

Servings: 12

Ingredients:

- 200g oats
- 250g buckwheat flakes
- 100g walnuts, chopped
- 100g almonds, chopped
- 100g dried strawberries
- 1 ½ tsp ground ginger
- 1 ½ tsp ground cinnamon
- 120mls olive oil
- 2 tbsp. honey

Directions:

1. Preheat oven to 150C or gas mark 3. Line a tray with baking parchment.
2. Stir together walnuts, almonds, buckwheat flakes and oats with ginger and cinnamon. In a large pan, warm olive oil and honey, heating until the honey has dissolved.
3. Pour the honey-oil over the other ingredients, stirring to ensuring an even coating. Separate the granola evenly over the lined baking tray and roast for 50 minutes, or until golden.
4. Remove from the oven and leave to cool. Once cooled add the berries and store in an airtight container. Eat dry or with milk and yogurt. It stays fresh for up to 1 week.

Nutrition: Calories: 178 kcal Protein: 6.72 g Fat: 10.93 g Carbohydrates: 22.08 g

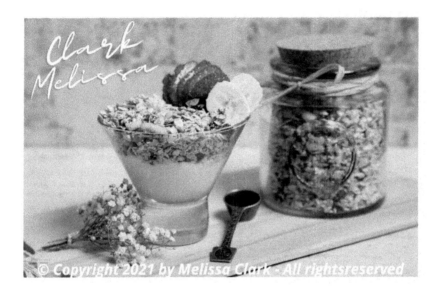

Tomato Frittata

Preparation Time: 55 minutes

Cooking Time: 20 minutes

Servings: 2

Ingredients:

- 50g cheddar cheese, grated
- 75g Kalamata olives, pitted and halved
- 8 cherry tomatoes, halved
- 4 large eggs
- 1 tbsp. fresh parsley, chopped
- 1 tbsp. fresh basil, chopped
- 1 tbsp. olive oil

Directions:

1. Whisk eggs together in a large mixing bowl. Toss in the parsley, basil, olives, tomatoes and cheese, stirring thoroughly.
2. In a small skillet, heat the olive oil over high heat. Pour in the frittata mixture and cook for 5-10 minutes, or set. Remove the skillet from the hob and place under the grill for 5 minutes, or until firm and set. Divide into portions and serve immediately.

Nutrition: Calories: 269 kcal Protein: 9.23 g Fat: 23.76 g Carbohydrates: 5.49 g

Horseradish Flaked Salmon Fillet & Kale

Preparation Time: 55 minutes

Cooking Time: 30 minutes

Servings: 2

Ingredients:

- 200g skinless, boneless salmon fillet
- 50g green beans
- 75g kale
- 1 tbsp. extra virgin olive oil
- ½ garlic clove, crushed
- 50g red onion, chopped
- 1 tbsp. fresh chives, chopped
- 1 tbsp. freshly chopped flat-leaf parsley
- 1 tbsp. low fat crème fraiche
- 1tbsp horseradish sauce
- Juice of ¼ lemons
- A pinch of salt and pepper

Directions:

1. Preheat the grill.
2. Sprinkle a salmon fillet with salt and pepper. Place under the grill for 10-15 minutes. Flake and set aside.
3. Using a steamer, cook the kale and green beans for 10 minutes.

4. In a skillet, warm the oil over a high heat. Add garlic and red onion and fry for 2-3 minutes. Toss in the kale and beans, and then cook for 1-2 minutes more.

5. Mix the chives, parsley, crème fraiche, horseradish, lemon juice and flaked salmon.

6. Serve the kale and beans topped with the dressed flaked salmon.

Nutrition: Calories: 206 kcal Protein: 26.7 g Fat: 6.5 g Carbohydrates: 11.12 g

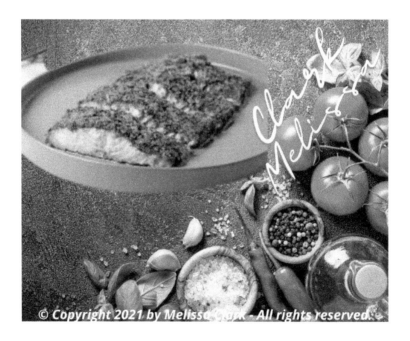

Sirtfood Scrambled Eggs

Preparation Time: 30 minutes

Cooking Time: 10 minutes

Servings: 1

Ingredients:

- 1 tsp extra virgin olive oil
- 20g red onion, finely chopped
- ½ bird's eye chili, finely chopped
- 3 medium eggs
- 50ml milk
- 1 tsp ground turmeric
- 5g parsley, finely chopped

Directions:

1. In a skillet, heat the oil over a high heat. Toss in the red onion and chili, frying for 2-3 minutes.

2. In a large bowl, whisk together the milk, parsley, eggs and turmeric. Pour into the skillet and lower to medium heat. Cook for 3 to 5 minutes, scrambling the mixture as you do with a spoon or spatula. Serve immediately.

Nutrition: Calories: 224 kcal Protein: 17.2 g Fat: 14.63 g Carbohydrates: 4.79 g

Chicken Thighs with Creamy Tomato Spinach Sauce

Preparation Time: 45 minutes

Cooking Time: 10 minutes

Servings: 2

Ingredients:

- One tablespoon olive oil
- 1.5 lb. chicken thighs, boneless skinless
- 1/2 teaspoon salt
- 1/4 teaspoon pepper
- 8 Oz tomato sauce
- Two garlic cloves
- 1/2 cup overwhelming cream
- 4 Oz new spinach
- Four leaves fresh basil (or utilize 1/4 teaspoon dried basil)

Directions:

1. The most effective method to cook boneless skinless chicken thighs in a skillet: In a much skillet heat olive oil on medium warmth. Boneless chicken with salt and pepper. Add top side down to the hot skillet. Cook for 5 minutes on medium heat, until the high side, is pleasantly burned. Flip over to the opposite side and heat for five additional minutes on medium heat. Expel the chicken from the skillet to a plate. Step by step instructions to make creamy tomato basil sauce: To the equivalent, presently void skillet, include tomato sauce, minced garlic, and substantial cream. Bring to bubble and

mix. Lessen warmth to low stew. Include new spinach and new basil. Mix until spinach withers and diminish in volume. Taste the sauce and include progressively salt and pepper, if necessary. Include back cooked boneless skinless chicken thighs, increment warmth to medium.

Nutrition: Calories: 1061 kcal Protein: 66.42 g Fat: 77.08 g Carbohydrates: 29.51 g

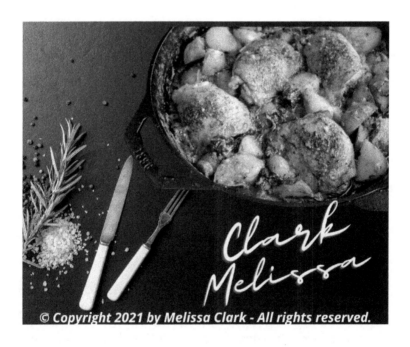

Creamy Beef and Shells

Preparation Time: 45 minutes

Cooking Time: 20 minutes

Servings: 2

Ingredients:

- 8 ounces medium pasta shells
- One tablespoon olive oil
- 1-pound ground meat
- One little sweet onion (diced)
- Five cloves garlic (minced)
- One teaspoon Italian flavoring
- One teaspoon dried parsley
- 1/2 teaspoon dried oregano
- 1/2 teaspoon smoked paprika
- Two tablespoons generally useful flour
- 1 cup meat stock
- 1 (15oz can) marinara sauce
- 3/4 cup overwhelming cream
- 1/4 cup sharp cream
- Legitimate salt and crisply ground dark pepper (to taste)
- 1/2 cups cheddar (newly ground)

Directions:

1. Cook pasta as per bundle directions in an enormous pot of bubbling salted water and channel well. Put an olive oil in a large skillet over medium-high warmth. Include ground meat and cook until caramelized, around 3-5 minutes,

breaking it with a wooden spoon. Channel abundance fat and put in a safe spot. To a similar skillet, include diced onion, and cook for 2minutes, mixing now and again. Include garlic, and cook until fragrant, around one moment. Speed in flour until delicately caramelized, for around one moment. Step by step rush in hamburger stock and mix to join. Include marinara sauce and mix in Italian flavoring, dried parsley, oregano, and paprika. Heat to the boiling point, diminish warmth and stew, mixing once in a while until decreased and somewhat thickened around 6-8 minutes. Mix in cooked pasta, include back meat. Mix in overwhelming cream until warmed through, about 1-2 minutes. Taste and change for salt and pepper. Mix in sour cream. Mix in cheddar until liquefied, about 1-2 minutes. Serve promptly, embellish with parsley whenever wanted.

Nutrition: Calories: 1196 kcal Protein: 81.68 g Fat: 61.32 g Carbohydrates: 88.46 g

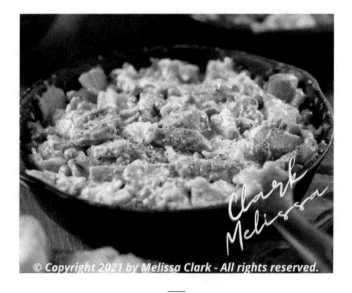

22

Shrimp Pasta

Preparation Time: 45 minutes

Cooking Time: 10 minutes

Servings: 2

Ingredients:

- 8 ounces linguine
- 1/4 cup mayonnaise
- 1/4 cup bean stew glue
- Two cloves garlic, squashes
- 1/2-pound shrimp, stripped
- One teaspoon salt
- 1/2 teaspoon cayenne pepper
- One teaspoon garlic powder
- One tablespoon vegetable oil
- One lime, squeezed
- 1/4 cup green onion, slashed
- 1/4 cup cilantro, minced
- Red bean stew chips, for embellish

Directions:

1. Cook pasta still somewhat firm as per box guidelines. In a little bowl, consolidate mayonnaise, stew glue and garlic. Race to join. Put in a safe spot. In a blending bowl, include shrimp, salt, cayenne and garlic powder. Mix to cover shrimp. Oil in a heavy skillet over medium warmth. Include shrimp and cook for around 2 minutes at that point flip and cook for an extra 2 minutes. Add pasta and sauce to the dish. Mood killer the warmth and combine until the pasta is covered. Include lime,

green onions and cilantro, and topped with red bean stew pieces.

Nutrition: Calories: 283 kcal Protein: 25.75 g Fat: 18.04 g Carbohydrates: 6.07 g

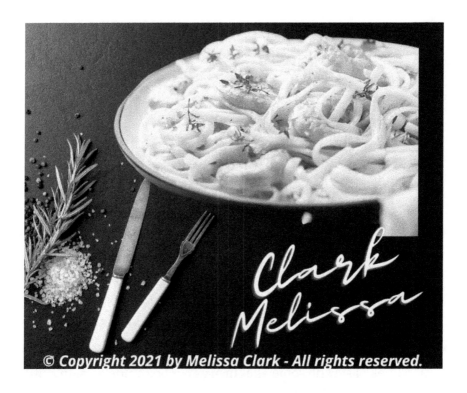

Lunch Recipes

Blueberry banana Pancakes with Chunky Apple Compote and Golden Turmeric Latte

Preparation Time: 5 minutes
Cooking Time: 30 minutes
Servings: 4
Ingredients:
For the Blueberry Banana Pancakes

- Six bananas
- 1 Six eggs
- 150g rolled oats
- 2 tsp baking powder
- ¼ teaspoon salt
- 25g blueberries

For the Chunky Apple Compote

- 12 apples
- 5 dates (pitted)
- 1 tablespoon lemon juice
- 1/4 teaspoon cinnamon powder
- Pinch salt

For the Golden Turmeric Latte

- 3 cups coconut milk
- 1 teaspoon turmeric powder
- 1 teaspoon cinnamon powder
- 1 teaspoon raw honey
- Pinch of black pepper (increases absorption)
- A tiny piece of fresh, peeled ginger root
- Pinch of cayenne pepper (optional)

Directions:

For the Blueberry Banana Pancakes

1. Pop the rolled oats in a high-speed blender and pulse for 1 minute or until an oat flour has formed.

(Tip: make sure your blender is very dry before doing this or else everything will become soggy!)

2. Now add the bananas, eggs, baking powder and salt to the blender and pulse for 2 minutes until a smooth batter form.

3. Transfer the mixture to a large bowl and fold in the blueberries. Leave to rest for 10 minutes whilst the baking powder activates.

4. To make your pancakes, add a dollop of butter (this helps to make them really delicious and crispy!) to your frying pan on medium-high heat. Add a few spoons of the blueberry pancake mix and fry for until nicely golden on the bottom side. Toss the pancake to fry the other side.

Nutrition: 394 calories

Savoury Turmeric Pancakes with Lemon Yogurt Sauce

Preparation Time: 5 minutes

Cooking Time: 20 minutes

Servings: 8

Ingredients:

For the Yogurt Sauce

- 1 cup plain Greek yoghurt
- 1 garlic clove, minced
- 1 to 2 tablespoons lemon juice (from 1 lemon), to taste
- ¼ teaspoon ground turmeric
- Ten fresh minutest leaves, minced
- 2 teaspoons lemon zest (from 1 lemon)

For Pancakes:

- Two teaspoons ground turmeric
- 1½ teaspoons ground cumin
- 1 teaspoon salt
- 1 teaspoon ground coriander
- ½ teaspoon garlic powder
- ½ teaspoon freshly ground black pepper
- 1 head broccoli, cut into florets
- 3 large eggs, lightly beaten
- 2 tablespoons plain unsweetened almond milk
- 1 cup almond flour
- 4 teaspoons of coconut oil

Directions:

1. Make the yogurt sauce. Combine the yogurt, garlic, lemon juice, turmeric, minutest and zest in a bowl. Taste and season with more lemon juice, if needed. Set aside or refrigerate until ready to serve.

2. Make the pancakes. In a small bowl, combine the turmeric, cumin, salt, coriander, garlic and pepper.

3. Place the broccoli in a food processor, and pulse until the florets are broken up into small pieces. Transfer the broccoli to a large bowl and add the eggs, almond milk, and almond flour. Stir in the spice mix and combine well.

4. Heat 1 teaspoon of the coconut oil in a nonstick pan over medium-low heat. Pour ¼ cup batter into the skillet. Cook the pancake until small bubbles begin to appear on the surface and the bottom is golden brown, 2 to 3 minutes. Flip over and cook the pancake for 2 to 3 minutes more. To keep warm, transfer the cooked pancakes to an oven-safe dish and place in a 200°F oven.

5. Continue making the remaining 3 pancakes, using the remaining oil and batter.

Nutrition: Calories 220

Sirt Chili Con Carne

Preparation Time: 10 minutes

Cooking Time: 10 minutes

Servings: 4

Ingredients:

- 1 red onion, finely chopped
- 2 garlic cloves, finely chopped
- 2 bird's eye chilies, finely chopped
- 1 tbsp. extra virgin olive oil
- 1 tbsp. ground cumin
- 1 tbsp. ground turmeric
- 400g lean minced Beef (5 per cent fat)
- 150ml red wine
- 1 red pepper, cored, seeds removed and cut into bite-sized pieces
- 2 x 400g tins chopped tomatoes
- 1 tbsp. tomato purée
- 1 tbsp. cocoa powder
- 150g tinned kidney beans
- 300ml beef stock
- 5g coriander, chopped
- 5g parsley, chopped
- 160g buckwheat

Directions:

1. In a casserole, fry the onion, garlic and chili in the oil. Over a medium heat for 2-3 minutes. Then add the spices and cook for a minute.
2. Add the minced Beef and brown over high heat. Add the red wine and allow it to bubble to reduce it by half.
3. Add the red pepper, tomatoes, tomato purée, cocoa, kidney beans and stock and leave to simmer for 1 hour.
4. You may have to add a little water to achieve a thick, sticky consistency.
5. Just before serving, stir in the chopped herbs.
6. Meanwhile, cook the buckwheat according to the packet instructions and serve with the chili.

Nutrition: Calories 267

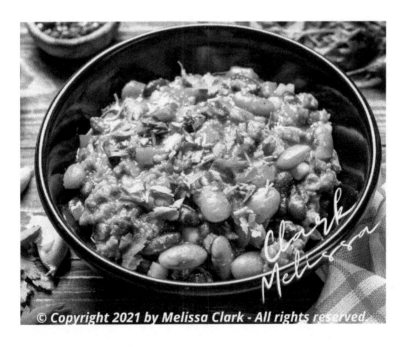

Buckwheat and nut loaf

Preparation Time: 15 minutes

Cooking Time: 30 minutes

Servings: 4

Ingredients:

- 225g/8oz buckwheat
- 2 tbsp. olive oil
- 225g/8oz mushrooms
- 2-3 carrots, finely diced
- 2-3 tbsp. fresh herbs, finely chopped e.g., oregano, marjoram, thyme and parsley
- 225g/8oz nuts e.g., hazelnuts, almonds, walnuts
- 2 eggs, beaten (or 2 tbsp. tahini for vegan version)
- Salt and pepper

Directions:

1. First of all, put the buckwheat in a pan with 350ml/1.5 cups of water and a pinch of salt. Boil it.
2. Cover and simmer with the lid on until all the water has been absorbed – about 10-15 minutes.
3. Meanwhile, sauté the mushrooms and carrots in the olive oil until soft.
4. Blitz the nuts in the food processor until well chopped.
5. Combine the vegetables, cooked buckwheat, herbs and chopped nuts and stir in the eggs. If using tahini instead of eggs combine this with some water to create a thick pouring consistency before stirring it into the buckwheat.
6. Season it with salt and pepper.

---

7. Transfer to a lined or oiled loaf tin and bake in the oven on gas mark 5/190C for 30 minutes until set and just browning on top.

Nutrition: Calories 163 Carbs 23g Protein 6g Fiber 4g

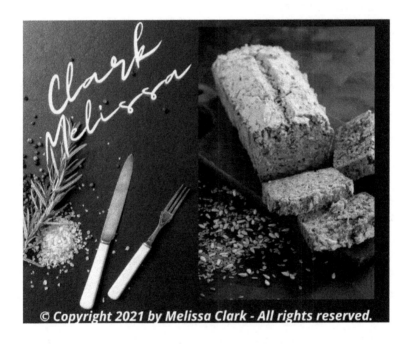

Quinoa Edamame and Pomegranate seed Pilaf

Preparation Time: 5 minutes

Cooking Time: 10 minutes

Servings: 4

Ingredients:

- ½ cup of sun-dried tomatoes
- 225g/8oz quinoa
- 1 cup of frozen edamame beans
- 2 tbsp. of hazelnuts
- 3 tbsp. olive oil
- 1 tbsp. lemon juice
- 2 tsp of tamari
- Salt and pepper
- 1 pomegranate
- 2 tbsp. coriander, chopped

Directions:

1. Put the sun-dried tomatoes in bowl. Cover with water and leave to soak. Now rinse the quinoa and put it in a pan with 350ml/11fl oz. of water and a pinch of salt. Boil it. Cover and simmer with the lid on until all the water has been absorbed – about 15 minutes.
2. Stir in the edamame beans.
3. Toast the hazelnuts in the oven for 8 minutes on gas mark 6/200C.
4. Drain the sun-dried tomatoes.

5. Combine the cooked quinoa with the sun-dried tomatoes and hazelnuts in a bowl.
6. Make your dressing by combining the olive oil, lemon juice and tamari. Gently stir this into the quinoa and vegetables.
7. Season it with salt and pepper and sprinkle on the pomegranate seeds and coriander.

Nutrition: Calories 236.6 Carbs 29.9g Protein 9.3g

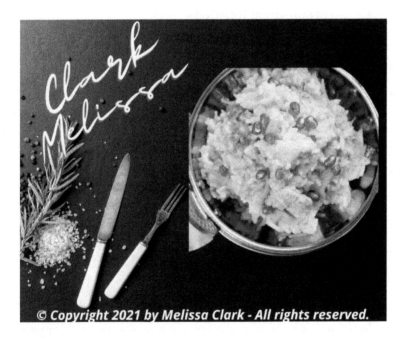

Sweet potato and salmon patties

Preparation Time: 10 minutes

Cooking Time: 20 minutes

Servings: 2

Ingredients:

- 225g/8oz wild salmon, cooked or tinned
- 225g/8oz sweet potato cooked and mashed
- Herb salt and pepper to taste
- Rice flour or buckwheat flour

Directions:

1. Preheat your oven to 160C/gas mark 3, then mix together the sweet potato, salmon, herb salt and pepper. Take a small handful of the mixture, roll it into a ball shape. Flatten it into a burger shape then dip each side in the flour. Place on a lined baking tray. Repeat until you have used up the mixture.

Nutrition: Calories 116 Carbs 13g Fat 2g Protein 9g

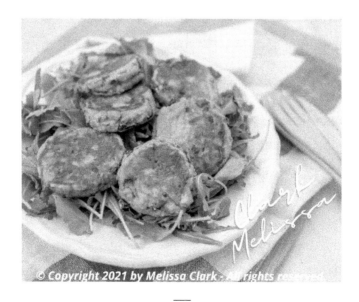

Moong Dahl

Preparation Time: 10 minutes

Cooking Time: 10 minutes

Servings: 4-6

Ingredients:

- 300g/10oz split mung beans (moong dahl)
- Preferably soaked for a few hours
- 600ml/1pt of water
- 2 tbsp./30g olive oil, butter or ghee
- 1 red onion, finely chopped
- 1-2 tsp coriander seeds
- 1-2 tsp cumin seeds
- 2-4 tsp fresh ginger, chopped
- 1-2 tsp turmeric
- ¼ tsp of cayenne pepper – more if you want it spicy
- Salt & black pepper to taste

Directions:

1. First drain and rinse the split mung beans. Put them in a pan and cover with the water. Bring to the boil and skim off any foam that arises. Turn down the heat, cover and simmer.

2. Meanwhile, heat the oil in a pan and sauté the onion until onion gets soft.

3. Dry fry the coriander and cumin seeds in a heavy-bottomed pan. Fry until they start to pop. Grind them in a pestle and mortar.

4. Add the ground spices to the onions and also add ginger, turmeric and cayenne pepper. Cook for a few minutes.

5. Once the mung beans are almost done, add the onion and spice mix to them. Season it with salt and pepper and cook for a further 10 minutes.

Nutrition: Calories 347 Protein 25.73 Fiber 18.06

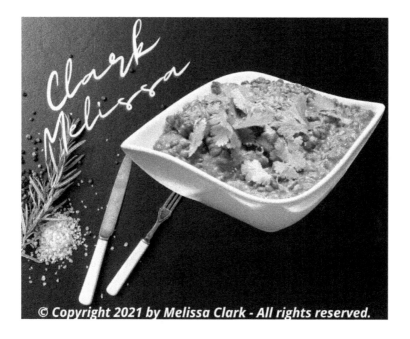

Almond Butter and Alfalfa Wraps

Preparation Time: 10 minutes

Cooking Time: 10 minutes

Servings: 3

Ingredients:

- 4 tbsp. of almond nut butter
- Juice of 1 lemon
- 2-3 carrots – grated
- 3 radishes, finely sliced
- 1 cup of alfalfa sprouts
- Salt and pepper
- Lettuce leaves or nori sheets

Directions:

1. First, mix the almond butter with most of the lemon juice and enough water to make a creamy consistency. Now combine the grated carrot, alfalfa sprouts in a bowl. Sprinkle them with the rest of the lemon juice and season with salt and pepper.

2. Spread the lettuce leaves or nori sheets with almond butter and top with the carrot and sprout mixture. Roll up and eat immediately!

Nutrition: Calories: 266

Aromatic chicken breast + kale and red onions + a tomato and chili salsa

Preparation Time: 15 minutes

Cooking Time: 20 minutes

Servings: 4

Ingredients:

- 8 tsp ground turmeric
- 480g skinless and boneless chicken breast
- 200 g of kale, chopped
- 1 lemon
- 4 tablespoons of extra virgin olive oil
- 80g of red onion, sliced
- 20 g of parsley, finely chopped
- 520 g of tomatoes
- 4 tablespoons of chopped fresh ginger
- 4 bird's eye chilies, finely chopped
- 4 tablespoons of capers, finely chopped

Directions:

1. Take out the tomato eye and chop it very finely,
2. Mix the tomatoes with the chili, parsley capers, and lemon juice. Preheat the oven to 220°C
3. Marinate the chicken breast using the lemon juice, 1 teaspoon of the turmeric, and a little oil. Leave for 5–10 minutes.
4. Heat the frying pan and place the marinated chicken in it. Cook for a minute on each side until it turns pale golden.

5. Transfer it to the oven and place in the baking tray for 8–10 minutes until cooked through.
6. Bring down from the oven and cover with foil. Allow resting for 5 minutes. Cook the kale for 5 minutes in a steamer.
7. Also, fry the red onions and the ginger using little oil to become soft, then add the cooked kale and continue to fry for another minute.
8. Cook the buckwheat according to instruction on the packet using the remaining teaspoon of turmeric.
9. Serve the chicken together with the vegetables and salsa.

Nutrition: Calories 340

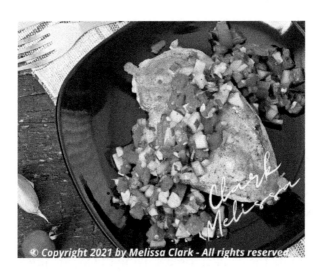

Fragrant Asian Hotpot

Preparation Time: 10 minutes

Cooking Time: 25 minutes

Servings: 4

Ingredients:

- 1 teaspoon of tomato purée
- ¼ teaspoon of star anise, crushed
- 10g of parsley with the stalk finely chopped
- 10g of coriander with the stalks finely chopped
- 1/2 lime
- 500ml chicken stock, fresh
- 1/2 carrot, peeled and sliced into matchsticks
- 50g of broccoli, diced into small florets
- 50g of beansprouts
- 100g of raw tiger prawns
- 100g of firm tofu, chopped
- 50g rice noodles, cooked
- 50g cooked water chestnuts, drained
- 20g sushi ginger, chopped
- 1 tablespoon of miso paste

Directions:

1. In a large saucepan, put the tomato purée, star anise, lime juice, chicken stock, parsley stalks, and coriander stalks, and simmer for 10 minutes.
2. Add the cabbage, pasta, water chestnuts, broccoli, prawns, and tofu to simmer till the prawns got finished.

3. Bring down from heat and add in the miso paste and sushi ginger. Serve mixed with the parsley and coriander leaves.

Nutrition: Calories: 262 Carbs: 21g Fat: 6g Protein: 24g

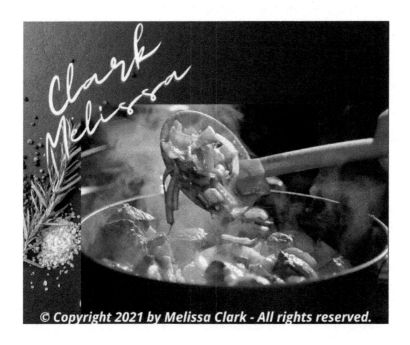

Greek Salad Skewers

Preparation Time: 10 minutes

Cooking Time: 30 minutes

Servings: 2

Ingredients:

- 2 wooden skewers
- 8 large black olives
- 8 cherry tomatoes
- 1 yellow pepper
- ½ red onion, chopped
- 100g cucumber, sliced
- 100g feta, chopped into 8
- Ingredients for the dressing
- 1 tablespoon of extra virgin olive oil
- ½ lemons
- 1 teaspoon of balsamic vinegar
- ½ clove garlic, peeled and crushed
- Few basil leaves, finely chopped
- Few leaves oregano, finely chopped
- Salt
- Freshly ground black pepper

Directions:

1. Soaked the wooden skewers into the water for 30 minutes
2. Thread each skewer with the salad ingredients in the order: olive, tomato, yellow pepper, red onion, cucumber, feta,

tomato, and olive, yellow pepper, red onion, cucumber, and feta.

3. Put the entire dressing ingredients in a bowl and mix together vigorously. Pour over the skewers.

Nutrition: Calories 236 Fat 46g Carbs 14g Protein 7g

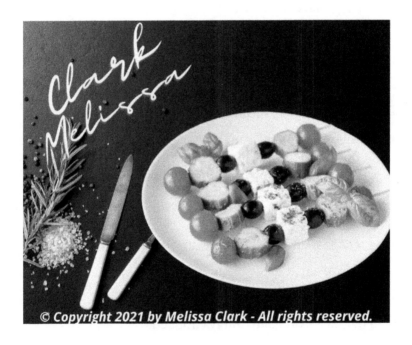

Dinner Recipes

Fried cauliflower rice

Preparation Time: 20 minutes
Cooking Time: 10 minutes
Servings: 4
Ingredients:

- 1-piece Cauliflower
- 2 tablespoon Coconut oil
- 1-piece Red onion
- 4 cloves Garlic
- 60 ml Vegetable broth
- 1.5 cm fresh ginger
- 1 teaspoon Chili flakes
- ½ pieces Carrot
- ½ pieces Red bell pepper
- ½ pieces Lemon (the juice)
- 2 tablespoon Pumpkin seeds
- 2 tablespoon fresh coriander

Directions:

1. Cut the cauliflower into small rice grains in a food processor.
2. Finely chop the onion, garlic and ginger, cut the carrot into thin strips, dice the bell pepper and finely chop the herbs.
3. Melt 1 tablespoon of coconut oil in a pan and add half of the onion and garlic to the pan and fry briefly until translucent.

4. Add cauliflower rice and season with salt.

5. Pour in the broth and stir everything until it evaporates and the cauliflower rice is tender.

6. Take the rice out of the pan and set it aside.

7. Melt the rest of the coconut oil in the pan and add the remaining onions, garlic, ginger, carrots and peppers.

8. Fry for a few minutes until the vegetables are tender. Season them with a little salt.

9. Add the cauliflower rice again, heat the whole dish and add the lemon juice.

10. Garnish with pumpkin seeds and coriander before serving.

Nutrition: Carbohydrates: 14g   Protein: 9g   Fat: 3g
Cholesterol: 47mg Sodium: 868mg Fiber: 6g Sugar: 1g

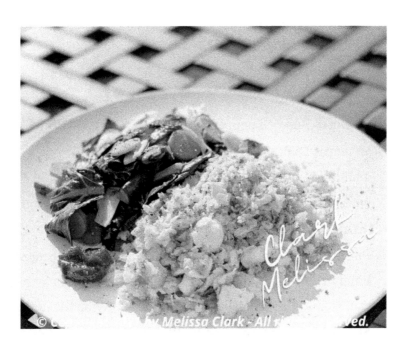

Fried chicken and broccoli

Preparation Time: 10 minutes

Cooking Time: 20 minutes

Servings: 4

Ingredients:

- 2 tablespoon Coconut oil
- 400 g Chicken breast
- Bacon cubes 150 g
- Broccoli 250 g

Directions:

1. Cut the chicken into cubes.
2. Melt the coconut oil in a pan over medium heat and brown the chicken with the bacon cubes and cook through.
3. Season it with chili flakes, salt and pepper.
4. Add broccoli and fry.

Nutrition: Calories: 308kcal   Carbohydrates: 15g
Protein: 37g   Fat: 12g   Cholesterol: 96mg   Fiber: 1g
Sugar: 6g

Mediterranean paleo pizza

Preparation Time: 20 minutes

Cooking Time: 25 minutes

Servings: 2

Ingredients:

- 2 tablespoon Coconut oil
- 400 g Chicken breast
- Bacon cubes 150 g
- Broccoli 250 g

Directions:

1. Cut the chicken into cubes.
2. Melt the coconut oil in a pan over medium heat and brown the chicken with the bacon cubes and cook through.
3. Season it with chili flakes, salt and pepper.
4. Add broccoli and fry.

Nutrition: Calories 274 Fat 17g Carbs 25g Protein 8g

Braised leek with pine nuts

Preparation Time: 10 minutes

Cooking Time: 20 minutes

Servings: 8

Ingredients:

- 20 g Ghee
- 2 teaspoon Olive oil
- 2 pieces Leek
- 150 ml Vegetable broth
- Fresh parsley
- 1 tablespoon fresh oregano
- 1 tablespoon Pine nuts (roasted)

Directions:

1. Cut the leek into thin rings and finely chop the herbs. Roast the pine nuts in a dry pan over medium heat.
2. Melt the ghee together with the olive oil in a large pan.
3. Cook the leek until golden brown for 5 minutes, stirring constantly.
4. Add the vegetable broth and cook for another 10 minutes until the leek is tender.
5. Stir in the herbs and sprinkle the pine nuts on the dish just before serving.

Nutrition: Calories 201 Carbohydrates 22 g Fat 12g Protein 2g Fat 3g Fiber 2g

Sweet and sour pan with cashew nuts

Preparation Time: 10 minutes

Cooking Time: 25 minutes

Servings: 2

Ingredients:

- 2 tablespoon Coconut oil
- 2 pieces Red onion
- 2 pieces yellow bell pepper
- 250 g White cabbage
- 150 g Pak choi
- 50 g Mung bean sprouts
- 4 pieces Pineapple slices
- 50 g Cashew nuts
- For the sweet and sour sauce:
- 60 ml Apple cider vinegar
- 4 tablespoon Coconut blossom sugar
- 1½ tablespoon Tomato paste
- 1 teaspoon Coconut-Aminos
- 2 teaspoon Arrowroot powder
- 75 ml Water

Directions:

1. Roughly cut the vegetables.
2. Mix the arrow root with five tablespoons of cold water into a paste.
3. Then put all the other ingredients for the sauce in a saucepan and add the arrowroot paste for binding.

---

4. Melt the coconut oil in a pan and fry the onion.

5. Add the bell pepper, cabbage, pak choi and bean sprouts and stir-fry until the vegetables become a little softer.

6. Add the pineapple and cashew nuts and stir a few more times.

7. Pour a little sauce over the wok dish and serve.

Nutrition: Calories 530 kcal

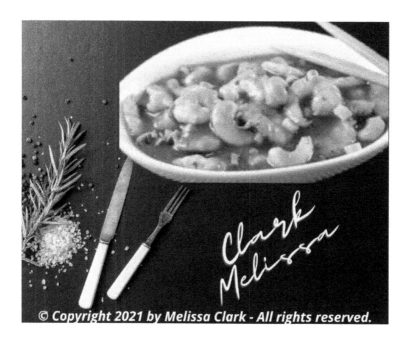

Casserole with spinach and eggplant

Preparation Time: 10 minutes

Cooking Time: 45 minutes

Servings: 6

Ingredients:

- 1-piece Eggplant
- 2 pieces Onion
- Olive oil 3 tablespoon
- Spinach (fresh) 450 g
- Tomatoes 4 pieces
- Egg 2 pieces
- 60 ml Almond milk
- 2 teaspoons Lemon juice
- 4 tablespoon Almond flour

Directions:

1. Preheat the oven to 200 ° C.
2. Cut the eggplants, onions and tomatoes into slices and sprinkle salt on the eggplant slices.
3. Brush the eggplants and onions with olive oil and fry them in a grill pan.
4. Shrink the spinach in a large saucepan over moderate heat and drain in a sieve.
5. Put the vegetables in layers in a greased baking dish: first the eggplant, then the spinach and then the onion and the tomato. Repeat this again.
6. Whisk eggs with almond milk, lemon juice, salt and pepper and pour over the vegetables.

7. Sprinkle almond flour over the dish and bake in the oven for about 30 to 40 minutes.

Nutrition: Calories 139.9 Cholesterol 72 Carbohydrate: 21.5g Protein 10.3g

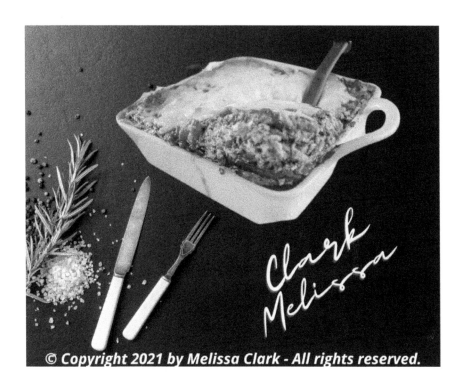

Vegetarian paleo ratatouille

Preparation Time: 20 minutes

Cooking Time: 1 hour

Servings: 4

Ingredients:

- 200 g Tomato cubes (can)
- 1/2 pieces Onion
- 2 cloves Garlic
- 1/4 teaspoon dried oregano
- 1 / 4 TL Chili flakes
- 2 tablespoon Olive oil
- 1-piece Eggplant
- 1-piece Zucchini
- 1-piece hot peppers
- 1 teaspoon dried thyme

Directions:

1. Preheat the oven to 180 ° C and lightly grease a round or oval shape.
2. Finely chop the onion and garlic.
3. Mix the tomato cubes with garlic, onion, oregano and chilli flakes, season with salt and pepper and put on the bottom of the baking dish.
4. Use a mandolin, a cheese slicer or a sharp knife to cut the eggplant, zucchini and hot pepper into very thin slices.
5. Put the vegetables in a bowl (make circles, start at the edge and work inside).

6. Drizzle the remaining olive oil on the vegetables and sprinkle with thyme, salt and pepper.

7. Cover the baking dish with a piece of parchment paper and bake in the oven for 45 to 55 minutes.

Nutrition: Calories 109 Carbohydrates 17g Fiber 4g Sugar 11g Protein 3g

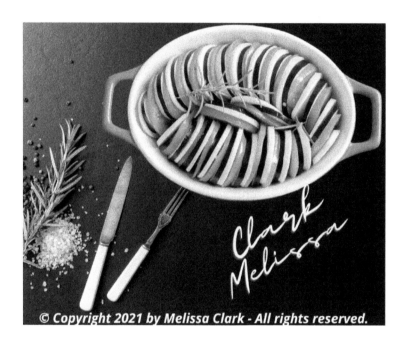

Courgette and broccoli soup

Preparation Time: 15 minutes

Cooking Time: 15 minutes

Servings: 6

Ingredients:

- 2 tablespoon Coconut oil
- 1-piece Red onion
- 2 cloves Garlic
- 300 g Broccoli
- 1-piece Zucchini
- 750 ml Vegetable broth

Directions:

1. Finely chop the onion and garlic, cut the broccoli into florets and the zucchini into slices.
2. Melt the coconut oil in a soup pot and fry the onion with the garlic.
3. Cook the zucchini for a few minutes.
4. Add broccoli and vegetable broth and simmer for about 5 minutes.
5. Puree the soup with a hand blender and season with salt and pepper.

Nutrition: Calories 115 Carbohydrates 17g Protein 5g

Frittata with spring onions and asparagus

Preparation Time: 10 minutes

Cooking Time: 25 minutes

Servings: 4

Ingredients:

- 5 pieces Egg
- 80 ml Almond milk
- 2 tablespoon Coconut oil
- 1 clove Garlic
- 100 g Asparagus tips
- 4 pieces Spring onions
- 1 teaspoon Tarragon
- 1 pinch Chili flakes

Directions:

1. Preheat the oven to 220 ° C.
2. Squeeze the garlic and finely chop the spring onions.
3. Whisk the eggs with the almond milk and season with salt and pepper.
4. Melt 1 tablespoon of coconut oil in a medium-sized cast iron pan and briefly fry the onion and garlic with the asparagus.
5. Remove the vegetables from the pan and melt the remaining coconut oil in the pan.
6. Pour in the egg mixture and half of the entire vegetable.
7. Place the pan in the oven for 15 minutes until the egg has solidified.

8. Then take the pan out of the oven and pour the rest of the egg with the vegetables into the pan.

9. Place the pan in the oven again for 15 minutes until the egg is nice and loose.

10. Sprinkle the tarragon and chili flakes on the dish before serving.

Nutrition: Calories 305 Fat 14.8g Sugars 4.8g

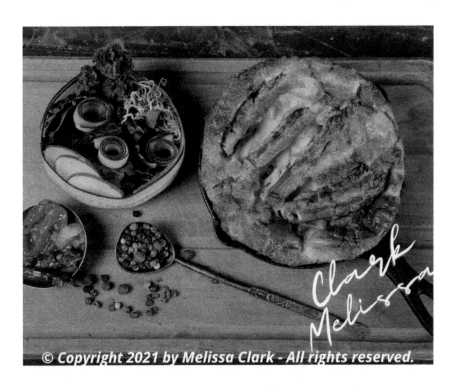

Cucumber salad with lime and coriander

Preparation Time: 10 minutes

Cooking Time: 10 minutes

Servings: 4

Ingredients:

- 1-piece Red onion
- 2 pieces Cucumber
- 2 pieces Lime (juice)
- 2 tablespoon fresh coriander

Directions:

1. Cut the onion into rings and thinly slice the cucumber. Chop the coriander finely.
2. Place the onion rings in a bowl and season with about half a tablespoon of salt.
3. Rub it in well and then fill the bowl with water.
4. Pour off the water and then rinse the onion rings thoroughly (in a sieve).
5. Put the cucumber slices together with onion, lime juice, coriander and olive oil in a salad bowl and stir everything well.
6. Season it with a little salt.
7. You can keep this dish in the refrigerator in a covered bowl for a few days.

Nutrition: Calories 104.2 Fat 7.2 Carbohydrate 6.4 Protein 2.2g

Appetizers & Snacks

Raw vegan chocolate hazelnuts truffles

Preparation Time: 10 minutes

Cooking Time: 30 minutes

Servings: 4

Ingredients:

- 1 cup ground almonds
- 1 tsp ground vanilla bean
- ½ cup of coconut oil
- ½ cup mashed pitted dates
- 12 whole hazelnuts
- 2 tbsp. cacao powder

Directions:

1. Mix all ingredients and make truffles with one whole hazelnut in the middle.

Nutrition: Calories 43 Carbs 21g Fat 4g Protein 6g

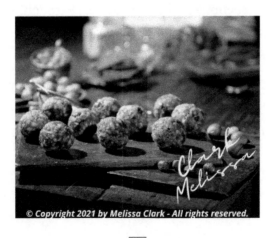

Raw vegan chocolate cream fruity cake

Preparation Time: 10 minutes

Cooking Time: 45 minutes

Servings: 4

Ingredients:

Crust:

- See Raw Walnut Pie Crust recipe
- Chocolate cream:
- 1 avocado
- 2 tbsp. raw honey
- 2 tbsp. coconut oil
- 2 tbsp. cacao powder
- 1 tsp ground vanilla bean
- Pinch of sea salt
- ¼ cup of coconut milk
- 1 tbsp. coconut flakes

Fruits:

- 1 chopped banana
- 1 cup pitted cherries

Top layer:

- Coconut whipped cream - see Coconut Whipped Cream recipes.

Directions:

1. Prepare the crust and press it at the bottom of the pan.
2. Blend all chocolate cream ingredients, fold in the fruits and pour in the crust.

3. Whip the top layer, spread and sprinkle with cacao powder.

4. Refrigerate.

Nutrition: Calories 123 Carbs 32g Fat 7g Protein 4g

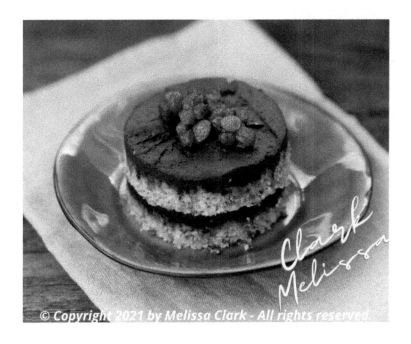

Raw vegan carob sesame truffles

Preparation Time: 10 minutes

Cooking Time: 35 minutes

Servings: 4

Ingredients:

- 1 cup ground walnuts
- 1 tsp ground vanilla bean
- ½ cup of coconut oil
- ½ cup mashed pitted dates
- 3 tbsp. carob powder
- 3 tbsp. chia seeds

Directions:

1. Mix all ingredients and make truffles.
2. Coat it with slivered almond or sesame seeds.

Nutrition: Calories 93 Carbs 32g Fat 1g Protein 8g

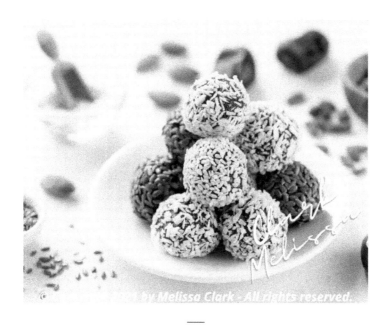

Snow-flakes

Preparation Time: 25 minutes

Cooking Time: 5 minutes

Servings: 6

Ingredients:

- Won Ton wrappers
- Oil to frying
- Powdered-sugar

Directions:

1. Cut won ton wrappers just like you'd a snow-flake
2. Heat oil when hot adds won-ton, fry for approximately 30 seconds, and then reverses over.
3. Drain on a paper towel with powdered sugar.

Nutrition: Calories: 191 Carbs: 20g Fat: 11g Protein: 3g

Lemon Ricotta Cookies with Lemon Glaze

Preparation Time: 15 minutes

Cooking Time: 15 minutes

Servings: 44

Ingredients:

- 2 1/2 cups all-purpose flour
- 1 tsp baking powder
- 1 tsp salt
- 1 tbsp. unsalted butter softened
- 2 cups of sugar
- 2 capsules
- 1 teaspoon (15-ounce) container whole-milk ricotta cheese
- 3 tbsp. lemon juice
- 1 lemon, zested

Glaze:

- 11/2 cups powdered sugar
- 3 tbsp. lemon juice
- 1 lemon, zested

Directions:

1. Pre heats the oven to 375 degrees F.
2. In a medium bowl, mix the flour, baking powder, and salt. Set aside.
3. From the big bowl, blend the butter and the sugar levels. With an electric mixer, beat the sugar and butter until light and

fluffy, about three minutes. Add the eggs1 at a time, beating until incorporated.

4. Insert the ricotta cheese, lemon juice, and lemon zest. Beat to blend. Stir in the dry skin.

5. Line two baking sheets with parchment paper. Spoon the dough (approximately 2 tablespoons of each cookie) on the baking sheets. Bake for fifteen minutes, until slightly golden at the borders. Remove from the oven and let the biscuits remaining baking sheet for about 20 minutes.

Glaze:

6. Combine the powdered sugar lemon juice and lemon peel in a small bowl and then stir until smooth. Spoon approximately 1/2-tsp on each cookie and make use of the back of the spoon to lightly disperse. Allow glaze harden for approximately two hours. Pack the biscuits to a decorative jar

Nutrition: Calories 131 Fat 3.7g Cholesterol 21.1mg Carbohydrate 22.3g Protein 2.5g

Clark
Melissa
© Copyright 2021 by Melissa Clark - All rights reserved.

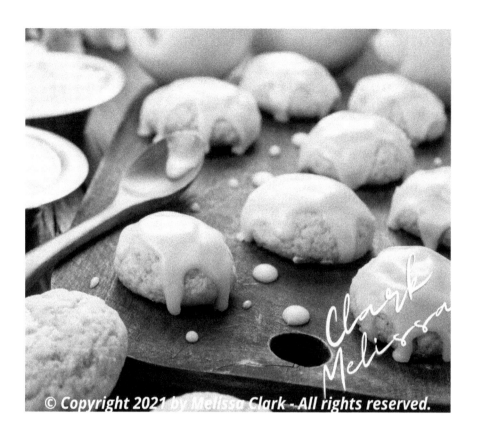

Home-made Marshmallow Fluff

Preparation Time: 10 minutes

Cooking Time: 20 minutes

Servings: 6

Ingredients:

- 3/4 cup sugar
- 1/2 cup light corn syrup
- 1/4 cup water
- ⅛ Tsp salt
- 3 little egg whites egg whites
- 1/4 tsp cream of tartar
- 1 teaspoon 1/2 tsp vanilla infusion

Directions:

1. In a little pan, mix together sugar, corn syrup, salt, and water. Attach a candy thermometer into the side of this pan, which makes sure it will not touch the underside of the pan. Set aside.

2. From the bowl of a stand mixer, combine egg whites and cream of tartar. Begin to whip on medium speed with the whisk attachment.

3. Meanwhile, turn the burner on top and place the pan with the sugar mix onto heat. Allow mix into a boil and heat to 240 degrees, stirring periodically.

4. The aim is to find the egg whites whipped to soft peaks and also the sugar heated to 240 degrees at near the same moment. Simply stop stirring the egg whites once they hit soft peaks.

5. Once the sugar has already reached 240 amounts, turn noodle onto reducing. Insert a little quantity of the popular sugar mix and let it mix. Insert still another little sum of the sugar mix. Carry on adding mix slowly, and that means you never scramble the egg whites.

6. After all of the sugar was added into the egg whites, then turn the rate of this mixer and also keep overcoming concoction for around 79 minutes until the fluff remains glossy and stiff. In roughly the 5 minutes mark, then add vanilla extract.

7. Use fluff immediately or store in an airtight container in the fridge for around two weeks.

Nutrition: Calories: 228kcal Carbohydrates: 58g Protein: 1g Sodium: 54mg Potassium: 68mg Sugar: 57g Calcium: 6mg

Clark
Melissa
© Copyright 2021 by Melissa Clark - All rights reserved.

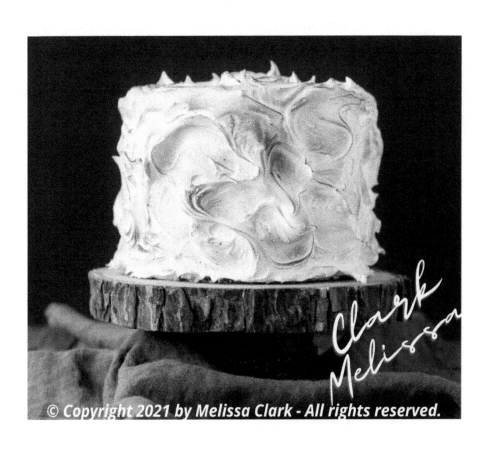

Side Dishes

Edamame

Preparation Time: 5 minutes

Cooking Time: 5 minutes

Servings: 6

Ingredients:

- 2 tablespoons sesame oil
- 1-pound edamame (frozen)
- 1 tablespoons chive (fresh, sliced thin)
- ¼ teaspoon red pepper flakes
- ½ teaspoon garlic powder
- 2 tablespoons sesame seeds
- ½ teaspoon salt (course)
- ½ teaspoon black pepper (ground)
- 1 cup water

Directions:

1. Pour the water into the inner pot of the Instant Pot, and then place a steamer basket in the pot.
2. Place the frozen edamame in the steamer basket.
3. Secure the lid, close the valve to sealing, select the steam option, and adjust the cook time to two minutes.
4. As the edamame steams, combine the chives, red pepper flakes, garlic powder, sesame seeds, salt, and ground black

pepper in a small mixing bowl. Mix together, and then set aside.

5. When the cook time is complete, carefully quick remove the lid.

6. Use oven mitts to lift the steamer basket out of the Instant Pot.

7. Transfer the edamame to a large mixing bowl.

8. Drizzle the sesame seed oil and add the chive mixture over top. Toss to coat evenly and enjoy.

Nutrition: Calories 170 Carbs 9.3g Fat 11.2g Protein 10.4g

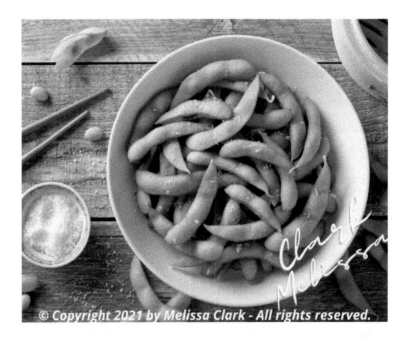

Hard-Boiled Eggs

Preparation Time: 1 minutes

Cooking Time: 5 minutes

Servings: for 12 eggs

Ingredients:

- 1/12 cups water
- 12 eggs (large)

Directions:

1. Pour the water into the Instant Pot and place the trivet inside. (You can place a steamer basket on top of the trivet or use the trivet to hold the eggs.)
2. Carefully arrange the eggs on the trivet or in the steamer basket.
3. Place the lid on, and set to sealing.
4. Choose Manual settings, set the cook time to five minutes, and then press start.
5. While the eggs are cooking, prepare an ice bath by adding ice to a bowl filled with water. Set aside.
6. When the eggs are done cooking, wait five minutes and then do a quick release by carefully moving the knob to venting.
7. Transfer the eggs to the ice bath.
8. Peel when ready to use. Serve in salad or as a side. Store it in the refrigerator.

Nutrition: Calories 126 Carbs 1g Fat 8.8g Protein 11.1g

Chicken Wings

Preparation Time: 5 minutes

Cooking Time: 25 minutes

Servings: 4

Ingredients:

- 4 ½ pounds chicken wings
- 1 teaspoon garlic powder
- ¼ teaspoon salt
- ½ teaspoon black pepper (ground)
- 1 cup water
- For the Buffalo Sauce:
- 1 cup hot sauce
- ½ cup butter (melted, unsalted)
- ½ teaspoon garlic powder

Directions:

1. Pour the water into the inner pot of your Instant Pot. Place the trivet inside.
2. Season your wings with garlic powder, salt, and ground black pepper. Place the wings on the trivet in the Instant Pot.
3. Secure the lid, turn the valve to sealing, select the manual setting, and set the cook time to eight minutes.
4. As the wings cook, combine the hot sauce, melted butter, and garlic powder into a large mixing bowl. Whisk thoroughly, and then set aside.
5. Once the cook time is up on the Instant Pot, let the pressure release naturally for 10 minutes. Then, carefully quick remove.

6. Remove the lid.

7. Use tongs to transfer the wings from the Instant Pot to the mixing bowl with the sauce. Toss to coat.

8. You can then place the wings on a baking sheet and place them in your broiler (high heat) to make the wings crispy. Broil them for five minutes.

9. Remove from the broiler and serve!

Nutrition: Calories 246 Carbs 2g Fat 24.5g Protein 6g

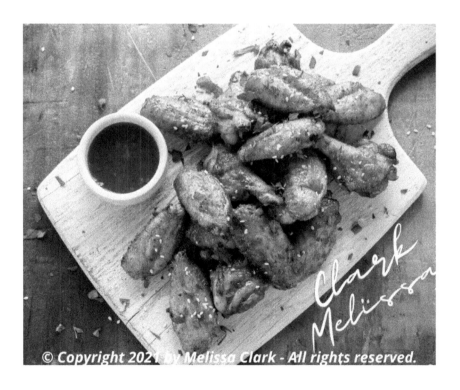

Chicken Dip

Preparation Time: 5 minutes

Cooking Time: 20 minutes

Servings: 8

Ingredients:

- 1-pound chicken breast (boneless, skinless)
- 1 ranch dip seasoning packet
- 1 cup hot sauce
- 1 stick of butter
- 16 ounces cheddar cheese (shredded)
- 8 ounces cream cheese

Directions:

1. Place the chicken breast, ranch seasoning, hot sauce, butter, and cream cheese into the inner pot of your Instant Pot.
2. Secure the lid, move the valve to sealing, select the manual option, and set cook time to 15 minutes.
3. When cook time is complete, carefully quick release.
4. Remove the lid. Take two forks and shred the chicken breasts.
5. Add the shredded cheddar cheese to the pot and stir.
6. Transfer the mixture to a serving bowl and serve with tortilla chips or crackers.
7. Store left overs in the refrigerator for up to four days. You can reheat it in the microwave or enjoy it cold.

Nutrition: Calories 302 Carbs 1.3g Fat 25.1g Protein 17.4g

Juices & Smoothies Recipes

Vegetable smoothie with banana

Preparation Time: 5 minutes

Cooking Time: 0 minutes

Servings: 1

Ingredients:

- 1 banana
- 1 hand kale
- 1 tbsp. unsweetened nut paste
- 1 date, seeded
- 100 ml unsweetened coconut milk
- 100 ml of water

Directions:

1. Get a blender; pour all the ingredients into it, and then blend.

Nutrition: Calories 177.1 Fat 3.8 g Sodium 40.8 mg Potassium 595.2 mg Carbohydrate 25.9 g Fiber 3.4 g Sugars 11.8 g Protein 13.4 g

Kiwi vegetable smoothie

Preparation Time: 5 minutes

Cooking Time: 0 minutes

Servings: 1

Ingredients:

- 1 kiwi
- 1 pear
- 1 hand kale
- ¼ avocado
- 1 date, seeded
- 100 ml unsweetened almond milk

Directions:

1. Get a blender; pour all the ingredients into it, and then blend.

Nutrition: Calories 105 Carbohydrates 22 g Protein 3.5 g

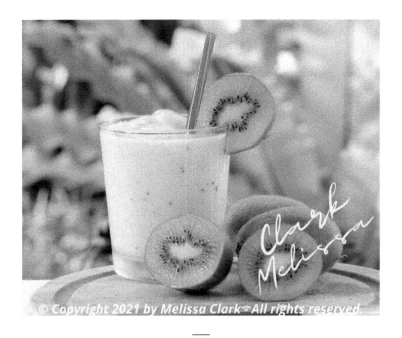

Cocoa smoothie

Preparation Time: 5 minutes

Cooking Time: 0 minutes

Servings: 1

Ingredients:

- 1 hand kale
- ¼ avocado
- 1 banana
- 75 g of blueberries
- 1 tbsp. (raw) cocoa powder
- 200 ml unsweetened almond milk

Directions:

1. Get a blender; pour all the ingredients into it, and then blend.

Nutrition: Calories 357.1 Protein 23.7

Clark
Melissa
Copyright 2021 by Melissa Clark - All rights reserved.

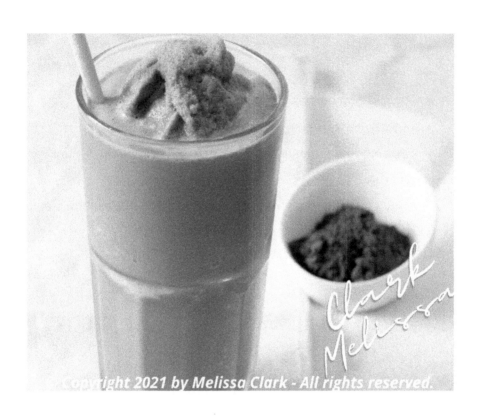

Pak Choy smoothie

Preparation Time: 5 minutes

Cooking Time: 0 minutes

Servings: 1

Ingredients:

- 4 stems bok Choy
- 2 peaches, seeded
- ¼ cucumbers
- 1 handful of cashew nuts
- 200 ml unsweetened almond milk

Directions:

1. Get a blender; pour all the ingredients into it, and then blend.

Nutrition: 9 calories 1.05 g of protein 1.53 g of carbohydrates

Endive smoothie

Preparation Time: 5 minutes

Cooking Time: 0 minutes

Servings: 1

Ingredients:

- 1 large hand endive (50 grams)
- 1 apple
- ¼ avocado
- 1 tbsp. linseed
- 1 tsp. (raw) honey
- 200 ml unsweetened almond milk

Directions:

1. Get a blender; pour all the ingredients into it, and then blend.

Nutrition: Calories 346.3

© Copyright 2021 by Melissa Cl

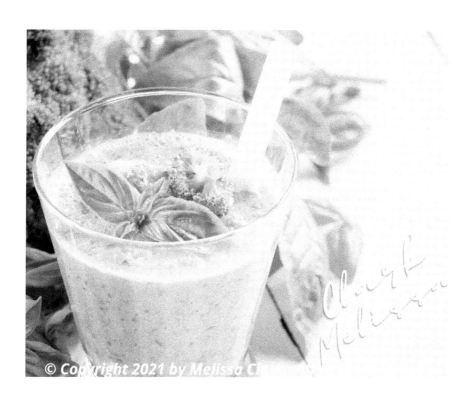

Coconut smoothie

Preparation Time: 5 minutes

Cooking Time: 0 minutes

Servings: 1

Ingredients:

- 200 grams of strawberries
- ½ bananas
- 1 hand endive
- 1 tbsp. chia seed
- 1 tbsp. coconut grater
- 200 ml unsweetened coconut milk

Directions:

1. Get a blender; pour all the ingredients into it, and then blend.

Nutrition: Calories 928.4 Sodium 59.6 Protein 9.4g

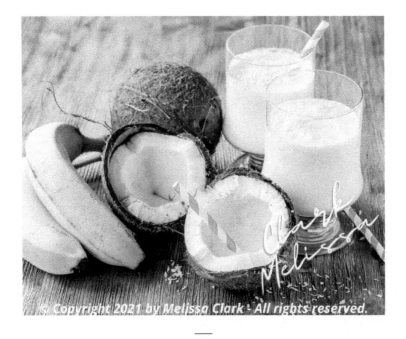

Yogurt smoothie

Preparation Time: 5 minutes

Cooking Time: 0 minutes

Servings: 1

Ingredients:

- 150 ml of Greek yogurt
- 125 g raspberries
- ½ bananas
- 1 tbsp. oatmeal
- 100 ml of water

Directions:

1. Get a blender; pour all the ingredients into it, and then blend.

Nutrition: Calories 121.7 Cholesterol 9.4mg Protein 7.5g

Clark
Melissa
© Copyright 2021 by Melissa Clark - All rights reserved.

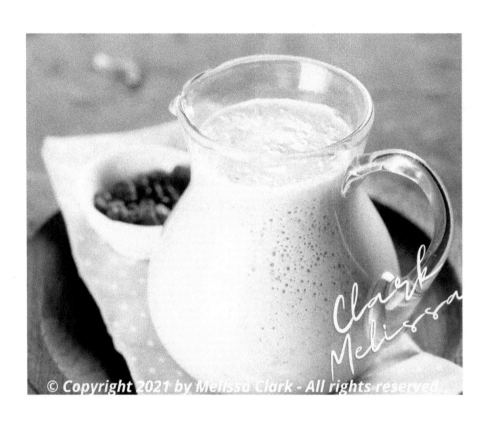

More Recipes

Mushroom tomato sauce

Preparation Time: 10 minutes

Cooking Time: 20 minutes

Servings: 6

Ingredients:

- 1 cup yellow onion, chopped
- 3 garlic cloves, minced
- 1-pound mushrooms, chopped
- 28 ounces tomato sauce, no-salt-added
- Black pepper to the taste

Directions:

1. Put the onion in a pot, add garlic, mushrooms, black pepper and tomato sauce and stir.
2. Cook over medium heat for 20 minutes
3. Leave aside to cool down.
4. Divide into small bowls and serve as a spread.

Nutrition: Calories 40 Carbohydrate 6g Protein 1g

Mulled Wine

Preparation Time: 10 minutes

Cooking Time: 20 minutes

Servings: 6

Ingredients:

- Dry red wine – 750 ml (1 bottle)
- Brandy – .25 cup
- Apple cider – 2 cups
- Honey – 3 tablespoons
- Cinnamon sticks – 2
- Star anise – 2
- Cloves, whole – 8
- Cardamom pods – 4
- Orange, sliced into rounds – 1

Directions:

1. Add all of the mulled wine ingredients into a large saucepan, stirring it to combine. Allow the wine to cook over medium-high heat just until it reaches a simmer. Don't allow it to boil, as this will cook off the alcohol.

2. Reduce the heat of the stove to low and cover the saucepan with a lid, allowing the wine to simmer to deepen the flavors. Simmer the wine for at least fifteen minutes, or up to three hours.

3. Use a fine mesh sieve to remove the spices and orange from the wine. Taste the drink and, if needed, you can add a little extra honey. Serve immediately while warm.

4. Sauces and Dips

5. While all of these sauces and dips may not contain the highest number of sirtfoods, that is okay! The point of these recipes is not to make up a large portion of your meal, but simply to add more flavor and variety to your food. With these recipes, you will find that the sirtfood diet can be diverse and flavorful, while also helping you to lose weight and gain health.

Nutrition: Calories 195

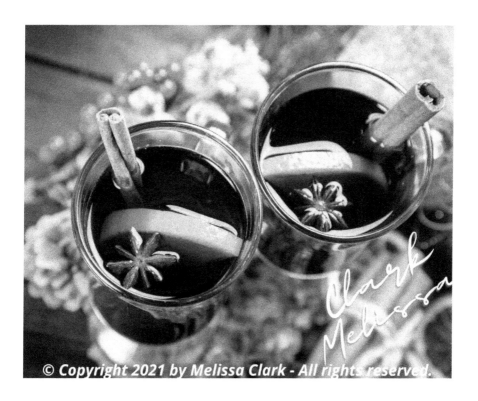

Sweet and Savory Cherry Compote

Preparation Time: 10 minutes

Cooking Time: 20 minutes

Servings: 6

Ingredients:

- Pitted sweet cherries, quartered – 2.5 cups
- Walnuts, chopped – 1 cup
- Red onion, diced – 2 tablespoons
- Extra virgin olive oil – 3 tablespoons
- Port red wine (or cherry juice) - .25 cup
- Sea salt - .25 teaspoon
- Honey – 1 tablespoon
- Rosemary, fresh – 1 teaspoon
- Black pepper, ground - .25 teaspoon

Directions:

1. Add the extra virgin olive oil into a large skillet and saute the red onion over medium heat until the red onion is soft and tender and beginning to turn golden around the edges, about three minutes. Be sure to stir the onions occasionally so the onion cooks evenly.

2. Add the cherries, walnuts, and rosemary to the skillet and continue to stir until the cherries become tender, about five minutes. Add in the seasonings and adjust the amount to fit your taste.

3. Pour in the red wine or cherry juice along with the honey. Allow the cherries to cook in the wine simmering slowly until

the cherries are soft and the liquid has become thick with a syrup-like texture.

Nutrition: Calories 240

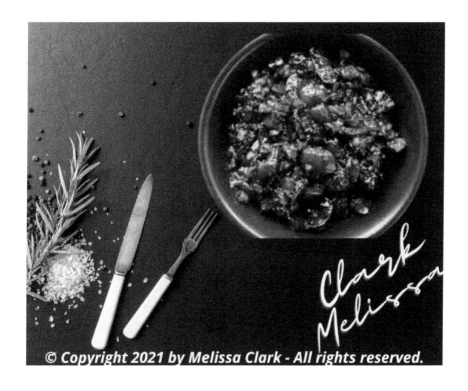

Cilantro Lime Sauce

Preparation Time: 3 minutes

Cooking Time: 3 minutes

Servings: 2

Ingredients:

- Soy yogurt, plain - .5 cup
- Black pepper, ground - .5 teaspoon
- Lime juice – 1 tablespoon
- Lime zest – 1 teaspoon
- Cilantro, chopped – 6 tablespoons
- Extra virgin olive oil - .5 tablespoons
- Sea salt .5 teaspoon

Directions:

1. Puree all of the cilantro lime sauce ingredients together in a blender or food processor until smooth. Serve the sauce immediately, or store in the fridge for up to a week.

Nutrition: Calories 71

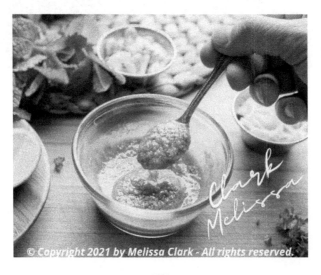

Greek Tzatziki Sauce

Preparation Time: 5 minutes

Cooking Time: 5 minutes

Servings: 12

Ingredients:

- Soy yogurt, plain – 1 cup
- English cucumber, grated – 1.5 cups
- Extra virgin olive oil – 1 tablespoon
- Garlic, minced – 2 cloves
- Lemon juice – 2 teaspoons
- Sea salt - .5 teaspoon
- Parsley, chopped – 2 teaspoons
- Dill, chopped – 2 teaspoons

Directions:

1. In a kitchen bowl whisk together all of the ingredients, excluding the cucumber.
2. Place the grated cucumber in a clean kitchen towel, and squeeze it over the sink to remove as much liquid as possible. Add the cucumber to the bowl, stirring it together to combine. Serve immediately, or store in the fridge for up to four to five days.

Nutrition: Calories 26

Green Enchilada Sauce

Preparation Time: 3 minutes

Cooking Time: 3 minutes

Servings: 6

Ingredients:

- Water - .5 cup
- Cashews, raw - .5 cup
- Cilantro, chopped – 2 cups
- Jalapeno, chopped – 1
- Green chilies, canned – 7 ounces
- Apple cider vinegar – 1.5 teaspoons
- Sea salt – 1 teaspoon

Directions:

1. Soak the cashews. To do this, either cover them with water or allow them to sit covered for six to twelve hours, or simmer them on the stove in water for fifteen minutes. Drain off the water and add the cashews to a blender.

2. Into the blender add the remaining ingredients and blend the enchilada sauce until it is completely smooth. Use the green enchilada sauce immediately or store it in the refrigerator for up to a week.

Nutrition: Calories 81

Jalapeno Pineapple Aioli

Preparation Time: 3 minutes

Cooking Time: 3 minutes

Servings: 12

Ingredients:

- Mayonnaise made with olive oil – 1.5 cups
- Onion, minced – 3 tablespoons
- Cilantro, chopped - .25 cup
- Jalapeno, minced – 1
- Canned pineapple, minced - .5 cup
- Garlic, minced – 1 clove
- Pineapple juice from can – 2 tablespoons
- Lime juice – 1 tablespoon
- Sea salt - .5 teaspoon
- Red pepper flakes - .5 teaspoon
- Lime zest – 1 teaspoon

Directions:

1. If you want a chunky sauce simply add everything to a bowl and stir it together.
2. For a smooth creamy sauce, pulse everything together in a blender until creamy.
3. Serve the jalapeno pineapple aioli immediately or store in the fridge for up to a week.

Nutrition: Calories 115

Awesome Sauce

Preparation Time: 5 minutes

Cooking Time: 5 minutes

Servings: 8

Time to Prepare/Cook: 5 minutes

Ingredients:

- Mayonnaise made with olive oil - .5 cup
- Sea salt – 1 teaspoon
- Mustard – 2 teaspoons
- Buffalo sauce - .5 cup
- Onion, diced – 1 cup
- Extra virgin olive oil – 1 tablespoon
- Parsley, chopped – 2 tablespoons
- Chives, chopped – 1 tablespoon
- Dill, chopped – 1 tablespoon
- Black pepper, ground - .25 teaspoon

Directions:

1. Add the onions and olive oil to a skillet, allowing them to saute until slightly translucent, about three minutes over medium-high heat.
2. In a blender, combine all of the awesome sauce ingredients, except for the chopped herbs. Continue to pulse until creamy, and then gently stir in the chopped herbs. Serve the sauce immediately, or store in the fridge for up to a week.

Nutrition: Calories 95

Vegan Hollandaise Sauce

Preparation Time: 5 minutes

Cooking Time: 5 minutes

Servings: 8

Ingredients:

- Mayonnaise made with olive oil (vegan) – 1 cup
- Lemon juice – 1 teaspoon
- Vegan butter, melted – 3 tablespoons
- Turmeric, ground - .5 teaspoon
- Cayenne pepper – .125 teaspoon
- Black pepper, ground - .25 teaspoon

Directions:

1. Add all of the vegan Hollandaise sauce ingredients to a small saucepan and cook it over medium heat until heated through. Be careful not to allow the Hollandaise sauce to boil.
2. Remove from heat and use hot. Enjoy the sauce immediately, or store it for up to a week.

Nutrition: Calories 177

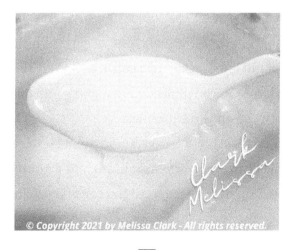

Vegan Cheese Sauce

Preparation Time: 5 minutes

Cooking Time: 5 minutes

Servings: 6

Ingredients:

- Yellow summer squash, sliced – 1
- Sweet potato, medium, peeled and diced – 1
- Garlic, minced – 4 cloves
- Onion, diced – 1
- Vegetable broth – 2 cups
- Nutritional yeast - .25 cups
- Sea salt – 1.5 teaspoons
- Mustard powder - .125 teaspoon
- Paprika - .25 teaspoon
- Black pepper, ground - .25 teaspoon

Directions:

1. Add the diced potato to a pot of boiling water, and allow it to boil until tender, about seven to ten minutes.
2. Meanwhile, saute the onion and yellow squash in the vegetable broth. Slowly add the vegetable broth as needed, using about one-quarter of a cup at a time and adding more as needed. Add in the minced garlic, and saute until it becomes aromatic, about three minutes.
3. Add the cooked onion, squash, and potato into a blender along with the remaining vegetable broth and all of the seasonings. Combine on high speed until the sauce is incredibly smooth.

Feel free to add more broth, to adjust the thickness to your preference.

Nutrition: Calories 57

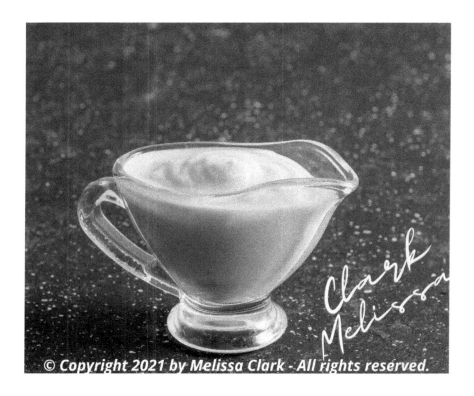

Easy Teriyaki Sauce

Preparation Time: 10 minutes

Cooking Time: 10 minutes

Servings: 6

Ingredients:

- Tamari sauce - .25 cup
- Water – 1.25 cups, divided
- Cornstarch – 2 tablespoons
- Honey – .25 cup
- Ginger, grated - .5 teaspoon
- Garlic, minced – 1 clove

Directions:

1. In a small bowl, use a whisk and combine together the one-quarter cup of water and cornstarch. Set the slurry aside.
2. In a saucepan add the remaining water along with the tamari sauce, honey, garlic, and ginger. While stirring, cook over medium heat until it reaches a simmer.
3. Add the cornstarch slurry into the saucepan while whisking, and continue to cook the sauce until thickened, about seven minutes.
4. Remove the easy teriyaki sauce from the stove and allow it to sit for five to ten minutes before using, to allow it to finish fully thickening.

Nutrition: Calories 57 kcal

Thai Peanut Sauce

Preparation Time: 3 minutes

Cooking Time: 3 minutes

Servings: 6

Ingredients:

- Peanut butter, natural - .5 cup
- Honey – 1 teaspoon
- Soy milk - .5 cup
- Tamari sauce – 2 tablespoons
- Ginger, grated - .5 teaspoon
- Lime juice – 1 tablespoon
- Sriracha sauce – 1 teaspoon
- Garlic, minced – 1 clove

Directions:

1. Add all of the Thai peanut sauce ingredients into a blender and combine until smooth and the garlic is well combined. Use the peanut sauce immediately or store in the fridge for up to a week.

Nutrition: Calories 138

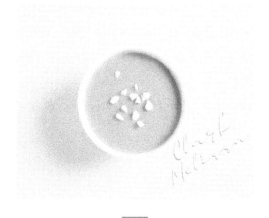

Milk of Gold

Preparation Time: 1 minute

Cooking Time: 4 minutes

Servings: 2

Ingredients:

- 250 ml of coconut milk
- 2 teaspoons of turmeric
- 3 teaspoons of honey
- 10 peppercorns
- The seeds of half a stick of vanilla
- Cinnamon

Directions:

1. Dilute the coconut milk with half a glass of warm water. Combine all the ingredients in a blender: diluted coconut milk, turmeric, honey, vanilla seeds and pepper crushed to the last.

2. Blend until you have obtained a well homogeneous and slightly frothy mixture.

3. Complete your golden milk with a sprinkling of cinnamon and serve by decorating with a whole cinnamon stick.

4. As an alternative to cinnamon, you can use star anise, blending it with all the ingredients and leaving it whole on top to decorate.

Nutrition: Calories: 205 Carbohydrates: 8.9 g Protein: 3.2 g Fat: 19.5 g

Spicy Eggs Mexican

Preparation Time: 10 minutes

Cooking Time: 5 minutes

Servings: 2

Ingredients:

- 4 eggs
- Peeled cherry tomatoes 500 g
- Butter 40 g
- 1 red pepper
- 1 clove of garlic
- 2 onions
- Red wine vinegar
- Red pepper
- Salt
- Pepper

Directions:

1. Peel the garlic and cut it into strips, then peel the onions and reduce them to veils. Put 374 of the butter in a pan and brown the garlic and onion for about 5 minutes. Add the pepper into chunks and let them dry for a couple of minutes.

2. Wet with a spoonful of vinegar, let it evaporate and add the chopped peeled tomatoes and the chopped chili pepper, then season with salt and pepper.

3. Cook for 45 minutes until you have a thick sauce. Heat the remaining butter and when it is melted, slide the eggs that you will have shelled into a plate. Cook over low heat until the egg white has not thickened, and the yolk will be liquid.

4. Salt, distribute the sauce in 4 bowls, put one egg in each and serve.

Nutrition: Calories 233 Fat 17.4g Carbohydrate 5.6g Protein 13.2g

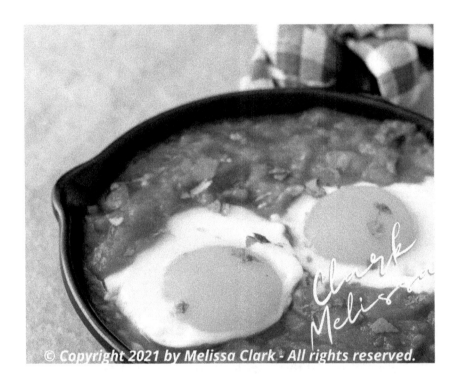

Waldorf salad

Preparation Time: 15 minutes

Cooking Time: 0 minutes

Servings: 4

Ingredients:

- 250 gr of celeriac
- 250 gr of apples
- 70 gr of walnuts
- 150 gr of mayonnaise
- 200 gr of yogurt (thick)
- 1 tbsp. honey
- 1 lemon
- Qs. of salt
- Qs. pepper

Directions:

1. To prepare the Waldorf salad, start cleaning the celeriac, peel it by cutting the peel with a knife, wash it and cut it into slices and then into strips.

2. Bring the salted water to a boil and blanch the celeriac for 2-3 minutes, then drain and pat dry with a tea towel. Now move on to cleaning the apples, wash them, peel them and cut them into slices and then into strips. Then dip the apples in water acidulated with lemon juice to prevent it from turning black (keep aside 1 tablespoon of lemon juice which you will need for dressing).

3. For the dressing, combine the mayonnaise, yogurt, a spoonful of lemon juice and honey, salt and pepper in a bowl, mix everything and add celery and apples.
4. Season the fruit and vegetables with the prepared dressing and add the coarsely chopped walnuts.

Nutrition: Calories 243 Fat 20g Carbohydrate 16g Protein 2g

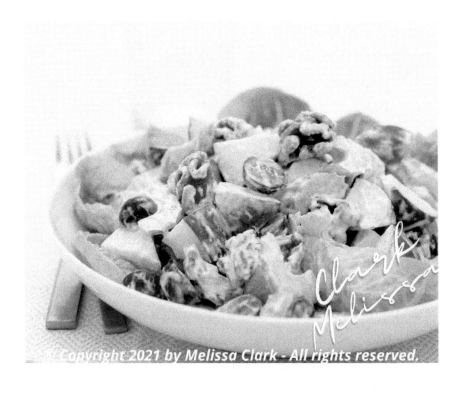

Brown Rice Salad with Octopus

Preparation Time: 15 minutes

Cooking Time: 60 minutes

Servings: 6

Ingredients:

- 500 gr of octopus
- 250 gr of brown rice
- 2courgette
- 1 clove of garlic
- 1 potato
- 1 egg
- Olive oil
- Salt
- Pepper

Directions:

1. First clean the octopus, then put it in a saucepan, cover it with cold water and put on the fire: cook for about 50 minutes after the boiling begins. Finally drain and let cool.

2. in the meantime, cook the rice, in abundant salted water, for the time indicated on the package, then drain it and let it cool too.

3. Cook the egg for 8 minutes from boiling to make it hard and boil the potato.

4. Wash and peel the courgette cut them into cubes and sauté them in a pan with a little oil and garlic. When they begin to soften, while remaining a little crunchy, add salt and pepper and let cool.

5. Cut the octopus into chunks, season it with salt, pepper, oil and parsley and add it to the courgette.

6. Also add the rice, the potato and the egg into chunks and gently mix everything.

7. Add potatoes and eggs.

8. Mix well.

9. Leave to rest in the fridge for 1 hour, and then serve your brown rice salad with octopus on the table.

Nutrition: Calories 154 Fat 7.6g Carbohydrate 18.8g Protein 2.9g

Clark
Melissa
© Copyright 2021 by Melissa Clark - All rights reserved.

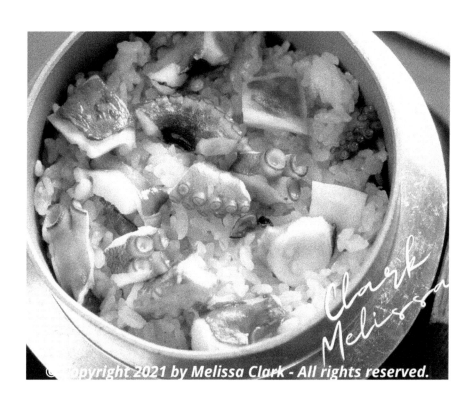

Conclusion

The plan will detoxify your body for seven days and then you'll need to keep eating sirtfoods to see the weight coming off, or you'll get it all back. This diet is not very healthy because, for most people, you're eating two of your meals, which isn't sustainable in the long term. It is a diet for those who are following a fantasy, and ready to pay for it. It is in no way resembles usual feeding and I assume it is unhealthy. It is very intense stuff.

Due to the high cost of exotic foods and the amount of time you'll spend juicing and cooking your meals, this diet will be incredibly hard to follow for many reasons. If you don't like matcha or kale then you'll find this diet very hard to follow as many of the Sirtfood Diet recipes contain both of these ingredients. Most people just flat out hated the way the drinks smelled, and couldn't even bother with the diet.

Throughout this book, you have not only learned the basic information required to start the Sirtfood diet, but you have also gained much more than that! By learning how to meal plan, prep, and storage, you will be able to easily master the Sirt food diet with little day-to-day effort required. You will be able to enjoy delicious meals at a moment's notice without having to struggle after a long day of work. By just preparing a little ahead of time, you can have a fridge and freezer fully stocked with delicious homemade meals perfectly suited to your taste.

The menu plan I provided you will help you get on your feet. Whether you choose to use the plan exactly how I designed, customize it, or create your own from scratch, you will find that by having a plan and guide to follow eating healthier, losing weight, and boosting your health can be easier than ever.

Whether you start out following the Sirt diet to the letter or simply experimenting and enjoying the dishes in this book, you are sure to experience benefits and fall in love with food all over again. What are you waiting for? With just a little effort and time in the kitchen, you can get on your way to success. This diet is certainly not for everyone, and it requires a lot of funds and energy to get through the meal preparation. The book includes several recipes about halfway through your reading, but many of the ingredients are so special that consumers found it hard to find them at the grocery store, as well as the tastes were so different in the beginning. Generally, this diet is backed by science, as many case studies have been shown, but for the average person, the possibility of seeing results from this diet alone is a long shot.

I hope you have enjoyed reading this book. More joy than sharing a healthy lifestyle, more balanced, and more enjoyable meal plan than the Sirtfood diet. I am sure you will enjoy all the fantastic recipes of this book.

Thank you
Clark
Melissa
© Copyright 2021 by Melissa Clark - All rights reserved.

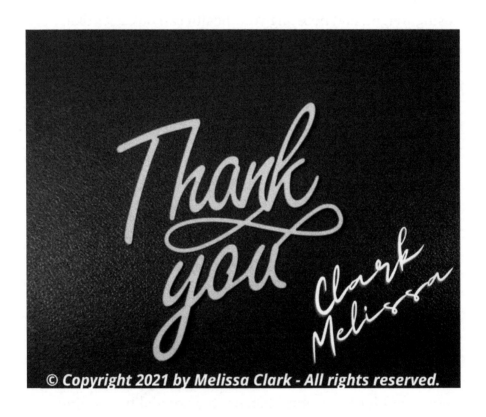

Lightning Source UK Ltd.
Milton Keynes UK
UKHW020037110321
380138UK00003B/328

9 781802 082227